Strategic Heart Failure

While every precaution has been taken in the preparation of this book, the publisher assumes no responsibility for errors or omissions, or for damages resulting from the use of the information contained herein.

STRATEGIC HEART FAILURE

First edition. September 20, 2020.

ISBN: 978-1393833543

Written by Marc Silver, MD.

Also by Marc Silver, MD

Strategic Heart Failure

Watch for more at StrategicHeartFailure.com.

Strategic Heart Failure

The strategies you, your family and your medical team should use to get you optimal heart failure care.

Marc A. Silver, MD, FACP, FACC, FAHA, FHFSA

Chandler, AZ

2020

Disclaimer

The information provided in this book is based on decades of experience providing care for patients with heart failure. It is intended to provide helpful information of the subject discussed. This book is not meant to be used, nor should it be used, to diagnose or treat any medical condition. Always consult your own physician and healthcare team. In fact, the information in this book is best used in collaboration with the members of your healthcare team and is intended to build a stronger more empowered relationship with them. The author is not responsible for any specific health or allergy needs that may require medical supervision and is not liable for any damages or negative consequences from any treatment, action, lack of action, application or preparation, to any person reading or following the information in this book. References, when provided, are provided for information purposes only and do not constitute an endorsement of any website, publication, organization or other sources. Readers should be aware that websites, when provided within this book, may change.

Dedication

The decision to write another book on the topic of heart failure is totally motivated by my desire, yet incomplete success, over a period of almost 40 years, to make sure patients and their families could all obtain optimal care and outcomes. The good news is that those 40 years provided me learning, wisdom and understanding.

But this book is not trying to pack all that learning into an expanded version of my prior books. Instead, Strategic Heart Failure is built around a few basic beliefs. One, the patient and family members must be partners in provision of their care. Two, understanding of a few fundamentals of care, especially the metrics and language that guideline directed care is crafted from, is totally within the grasp of patients and families. And third, the best care arises from caring teams welcoming in engaged and collaborative patients as partners.

Therefore, this book is dedicated firstly to all patients and families who followed the path outlined above with me for nearly 4 decades. They made my life richer and sweeter and more rewarding. I hope I gave them more life, enjoyment and empowerment to be my partner. Together we did the trial of what that partnership looks like-I call it **Strategic Heart Failure**.

It is also dedicated to my colleagues, my children and my dear wife Meredith. They have all, over the years supported me, tolerated me, challenged me, taught me and have done so graciously and with love.

As we say, success with heart failure.

Marc A. Silver

Chandler, AZ

2020

"Strategy is a fancy word for coming up with a long-term plan and putting it into action."

Ellie Pidot

"The essence of strategy is choosing what not to do." Michael Porter

"Success is 20% skills and 80% strategy. You might know how to succeed, but more importantly, what's your plan to succeed?" Jim Rohn

Table of Contents

Preface

This book feels very personal to me for many reasons. Dr. Silver and I cared for patients with heart failure when it wasn't "sexy" and when we had few options to offer. Together with others in our small but national interest group, we told stories of patients' symptoms, their journey and often frustrating outcomes. We formed friendships borne of our desire to do better for our patients. Subsequently and collectively, we navigated exciting times of discovery of successful treatments that both extended life and made its quality better. Our conversations with patients changed from "I can probably improve how you feel, but won't be able to stop the worsening of your condition" to "I can improve your symptoms and may be able to arrest the progression of your condition and extend your life—we now have treatments that work."

However, sometimes blinded by our own excitement and as pawns of a changing healthcare system, our patient visits became shorter. Our time for patient information sharing was markedly diminished while yet the interest in heart failure grew worldwide.

Nonetheless, in the midst of these changes and our own awe at new treatments, some things did not change: Our patients' symptoms and how scary hearing the words "heart failure" have meant to so many. Today, we use words that denote the patient as a true partner. A lovely thought that seldom becomes reality.

That is the starting point for this important book: Placing the patient in the driver's seat of their care. Using his incredible experience in heart failure care, Dr Silver has broken down the polyphony of terms that we often use among ourselves, into clearly understandable language. With this book, patients will better grasp our desire to practice by Guidelines and enter the conversation of what is best for them. Thus, a Strategic plan, not a haphazard one where crises rule the day.

It is my sincere hope that patients and caregivers come to view this book as their dictionary of heart failure care and that it emboldens them to enter the conversation as a true partner to get the care that they deserve. My congratulations to my friend Dr. Marc Silver!

Ileana L. Piña, MD, MPH, FAHA, FACC

Professor of Medicine Wayne State Univ

Clinical Professor of Medicine, Central Michigan University

Not angry...but frustrated.

This book is about you and your daily battle with heart failure. However, first, I think it is fair to let you know why I am writing this book. Any of you who have read my prior books (Success with Heart Failure) know that the first chapter in each edition was called Don't be Angry.

The reason for that was my understanding at the anger and fear and many other emotions patients and families struggled with trying to understand what heart failure was, where it came from, how it was changing their lives, how they felt, their financial future and even their survival. These strong emotions, while merited, often blocked their way to understanding and importantly, taking actions that they needed to learn, understand and get on top of this heart failure journey they were upon. I knew that blocking them from success were these emotions, along with depression and a condition that sapped their energy, limited their ability to read and understand complex instructions or medication changes, let alone grasp the continued bombardment of messaging they received when hospitalized, often from completely different teams every single day.

So, I wanted them to start at a place of greater calm, preparedness for learning and acknowledgement and acceptance about the emotions that are real, painful at times but also limiting.

And now, many years later I found myself looking back at the impact of my professional life's work exclusively in the area of heart failure. As many of you know from my bio (www.strategicheartfailure.com[1]) I tried to accept every opportunity to learn more, work to create scientific advances, publish and help others promote these advances, write guidelines so that others could learn about heart failure and measures that were indeed lifesaving. Mostly, my overriding emotion throughout my career was pride and joy. I was fortunate enough to have taken an interest in heart failure at a time when few others cared to. And over the subsequent years amazing advances were made with medical and surgical care to the point of having a large enough body of scientific data that the American

---

1. http://www.strategicheartfailure.com

Board of Internal Medicine created a new Fellowship level exclusively for Advanced Heart Failure and Transplant Medicine.

Yet despite my pride and joy, I also had other emotions triggered by our ability as a medical community to stem the tide of the heart failure epidemic. For all the effort, attention and advances it seemed like heart failure care was not advancing, huge gaps existed in care and outcomes and no one seemed to understand why. Even worse, it seemed to me that the plan, basically, was more of what we had been doing for decades.

For me, aware of how the emotion of anger could sidetrack all good work and intentions I was committed to not succumb to anger. However, I was, at the very least, frustrated.

The solution for my own personal frustrations with the gaps in care and outcomes for the millions of patients with heart failure, and the millions more in the early stages and headed directly into the same gaps in care prompted me to look at my personal experiences with the patients care for within our skilled team and other wonderful teams across the country. None of us had special tools or wisdom. Somehow, though our patients had a plan, and it was a plan crafted and followed by every member of the team. This was not done without effort; however, the planning and thinking that went into crafting the course for each patient, even before we made a single change in a medication seemed to be part of the secret sauce. That along with compassion, understanding, communication, repeated review of what we know about the patient, and gap filling at every visit, phone call or encounter seemed to be what made it work for our patients. And in the end the patients, their families and our team carried our overall pride and joy into this very specific work which lead to better outcomes and survivals.

In truth, the concept of strategic heart failure came from one of my patients. When patients would come to see our team, they knew the process; we would talk with them, examine them, and then take a pause where we all thought silently about what we knew and what were the next possible best steps, or at least the options. I was like the part of a chess game between the 2 opponents moves. Our patients also knew that we would never leave the room until ALL of their questions were answered, and we made sure everyone knew and agreed upon the plan.

One time, a newer patient who was not yet familiar with this silent pause for "thinking" during the visit began to ask a question. One of the other team members was in the room at the time and said, "sshhh, he's thinking". I thought the patient might have been offended, but instead, having been in the military most of his career, he just smiled and said, "oh, he's creating his strategy".

That comment has remained with me from that time on. And, honestly, that was what we did as a team. As part of our process we started from a point of asking if everything was in perfect order and nothing more needed to be done. Since that was rarely the case, we then asked ourselves "what were we missing?" even to the smallest detail. If there was any gap in what was optimal for that individual patient we then asked, "is there any reason for not trying to fill the gap(s)?"

And so, it became this repeating process of continual improvement rather than accepting the status quo. What we also discovered was that once patients and families understood the process of "Strategic Heart Failure" management they provided more challenging situations to see if we could find a way to optimize them so they could do something important to them. I remember clearly a patient who had a tradition of camping and hiking in the Teton National Park each summer with his family. I had never been there but remember the gleam in his eyes as he used to describe the fun and beauty, he and his family had every year they returned. As also understood that this was a pretty active vacation for him and his family. When he first came to see us, he had pretty advanced heart failure. So, we applied the Strategic Heart Failure approach and he got considerably better. However, he had other issues with degenerative hips and knees and so lung issues. I presumed that his Teton memories were all he had at that point. Nonetheless, he asked if there was a way for him to take another summer trip to the Tetons. We crafted a strategy which was a several months plan of optimization that included a pretty rigorous physical training program, mostly aimed at re-conditioning his muscles so once there he could climb and hike—without those activities we knew the trip would be unfulfilling. Anyway, thanks to our combined teamwork and our strategy planning sessions he did return to the Tetons that year, and actually for 3 more years after that!

So, you see, this book really reflects an approach that I want to share with each of you and allow you to apply it to your heart failure care. It takes your involvement and engagement for sure. We often think that when we choose our medical team that is the end of our responsibility. We will leave in their hands since they are the doctors and nurses—they are the experts. And, indeed they are. However, they are also human, often overworked, often practicing in a pattern that they learned in training, often concerned about completing some new mandate or checklist, or focused on learning the new electronic medical record or dictation system are asked to use. I do not think a single one of them are disinterested or not compassionate. It is just that your heart failure is a 24/7/365 enemy—they are not and cannot be ever vigilant about you and may not re-think the options for you care until you next visit. So yes, Strategic Heart Failure does rely on technology and on compassion and advances and wisdom. It is really about how all those tools come together and with what frequency and with what goals. It is a framework for thinking and caring.

I hope that Strategic Heart Failure will become your next best friend!

How to Use this Book

One of the pieces of the Success with Heart Failure books that was very well received was my personal suggestions as to how best use or read this book. There is no single best way and obviously what works for you is the best for you!

It is important to know that the #1 focus of this book is getting you to understand and use this book and these materials to get you the very best heart failure care you can have. This is not a book that explains what heart failure is, the many causes, the various types of medicine, what is an echocardiogram, and so on. As I looked back on the Success with Heart Failure series those books did that pretty well and much of that information has not changed substantially. Those books remain available even at your own library and also so much more is available online at trusted educational sites on the web. That information you might call Heart Failure 101. It is the important but only introductory information about heart failure. Even mastering that information does not immediately translate into providing you with optimal care. This book and the masterclass, Strategic Heart Failure, is the advanced class and clearly relies on knowledge and understanding of the basics. So, if you just discovering heart failure, or this is a new diagnosis for you, or you are just getting referred to see a heart failure team, advanced heart failure or transplant team or you are completely terrified and bewildered by the whole heart failure world, I suggest you take quick review of material and resources that can get you up to speed and prepare you to get the most benefit from the Strategic Heart Failure materials.

However, here a few tips and pointers as you begin.

From this point forward the book is structured in a step by step approach that is a logical approach that facilitates it being strategic. For example, I will soon talk about the importance of knowing what type of heart failure you have, or its cause. I will also talk about what stage of heart failure you have. That makes sense before you would expect your team to know how to treat your heart failure, you would expect them to be really certain as to what you have and what category of severity it is.

Each chapter is a logical progression from one step to the next and each step built upon the all of the prior steps. I have to tell you that my father's favorite piece of advice was always that good decisions in life are always created "step by step"!

Some of the decision patterns are exactly that. Patterns of a few steps that are often repeated over and over again. Such as, the patient has more symptoms, leading to the question of whether there are gaps in their current medical treatment that can be improved upon, to making that change and observing the result. Ultimately, getting to target doses of all of the key medications or at least the doses that are optimal for each patient mandates this kind of repetitive pattern approach.

However, there are times when there is a single problem you might be experiencing that needs the teams focus. And you may have already heard a variety of opinions on what the next best step is to fill in that gap. An example might be that your team tells you that your increased fatigue may be due to a slow heart rate, and that is likely being caused by a medication that they want to reduce or stop. Another team member might tell you that the medication should not be stopped because it is a crucial medicine and a pacemaker is the best approach. And still another team member might suggest getting some repeat testing to make sure you get the kind of pacemaker most likely to benefit you in the long run.

These complex decisions often asking layers of questions, thinking beyond a simple reflex decision and truly getting consensus and adherence from most team member. This is strategic.

The book can also be used as a point of discussion with your team who, while well intended, may not always use this strategic approach. And for sure the book should be shared with family, friends, spouses and children so they can understand your role and the importance of their support and participation.

And the book contained limited pictures, diagrams, chart and tools but the few it does are critical parts of your knowledge base and should be referred to time and again.

There are many ways to use this book—-that said, let's get Strategic!

Name Your Heart Failure

So somewhere or at some time someone told you that you have heart failure or congestive heart failure or CHF. And who knows what you were told or what you heard next. Likely, what followed was a quick summary and then some discussion of what the medical staff was going to do for "your" heart failure. And, quite honestly, that is probably what you wanted to hear...what could be done to make your feel better and life longer.

However, for you and your team to truly create a strategic approach to your care, one that should endure for a lifetime of quality and continued improvement, using current knowledge and to do so stepwise so that no step limits the next possible steps. And it should be based on your goals and wishes—and you need to become an absolute key part of your medical team.

Obviously, if you find out you have heart failure suddenly and start your journey in a hospital or an emergency room, the priority will be providing you relief of your symptoms and initiating medical therapy. However, perhaps one of the very first steps you and your team should take is the carefully lay out all the facts that are currently in front of you. Obviously, more information will be added over time. However, wherever you are on your journey you should get a salad understanding of where your heart failure is and all of the facts that are currently available. This will drive that'll your understanding but also that the team.

Far and away, the most important part of this first phase of your journey every phase is construction of what I call the strategic heart failure patient profile tool. If you don't currently to have this at hand or in front of you then please go to the strategic heart failure website and download a copy of this free PDF file. (https://www.strategicheartfailure.com/index.php)

As you can see the very first items really deal with a description of what kind of heart failure you have. And since heart failure can be complex there are really multiple ways to describe what kind of heart failure you have. In the profile you'll see that the very first line is the word "etiology". This word means the cause or origin of a disease. For example, when healthcare professionals they go beyond just saying someone has pneumonia, they provide when they can the location, like right upper lobe or left lower lobe, its severity and the etiology or the presumed cause of the pneumonia, such as bacterial, viral, aspiration, etc. The importance is clear. The greater accuracy in defining the disease or the condition then the more accurate and specific the treatment will be, and hopefully the better the outcome for the patient. It often goes beyond that and that the treatment for one form of a disease turns out to be the wrong form of treatment for a different cause or etiology.

There are many, many forms of heart failure and so it gets described using multiple formats. However, when it comes to the etiology there are a handful of diseases or condition that can result in heart failure; many of these in the advanced phases of heart failure may look alike but the importance in knowing the etiology in treating the cause with the hopes of slowing or preventing progression to more advanced stages.

Some of the more common etiologies and their causes are:

Etiology Usual cause

Ischemic Blockage or arteries/heart attack

Hypertensive High blood pressure

Infiltration Substances such as iron or amyloid are

deposited in the heart muscle

Chemotoxic Damage from specific forms of chemotherapy

Familial Linked to a familial or genetic abnormality

We try to be as specific and accurate as possible and often getting a handle on the etiology is a

process that takes a while and involves rigorous testing.

Another term that is used, and fortunately less often than before is the word "idiopathic". This is

a fancy word that means we do not know the cause of the heart failure. As our testing evolves

and we are better at finding genetic causes for many more forms of heart failure we call

something idiopathic less often.

One interesting example is with a form of heart failure called hypertrophic cardiomyopathy. It i

a form of heart failure that has excessively thick parts of the heart along with issues with irregular heart beats, impaired blood flow from the heart and can be serious or even lethal. Because of the muscle thickening that predominates, it used to be called "IHSS" for idiopathic subaortic stenosis. Since those days we understand that most forms of this disease are actually genetic and there over multiple genetic variations that result in this disease. (See the discussion of the MOGES classification in Chapter 6).

Two other words you may hear are genotype and phenotype. These come from a growing understanding that many of the forms of heart failure have their roots in a person's genetic makeup. Other factors such as diet, alcohol and chemotherapy may impact the final form of their heart failure and even how they progress, which treatments are best and their prognosis. One way to think about these two terms is that the genotype is the "recipe"—the list of ingredients or instructions an individual's gene have encoded within them. The phenotype is how those gene express themselves, are influenced by other individual and personal features, and are, therefore, the final "cake or meal".

Other Important Ways to Describe Your Heart Failure Status

So, you now have a name to your heart failure. The next step is to do a careful self-audit on what symptoms you have, how limited (or not) you are by your heart failure and even do an honest review of how long you have had heart failure and what the progression has been. Often the disease sneaks up on you or commonly as your heart failure progresses you make subtle adaptations to what you do or how often or at what pace you undertake even daily activities. I know that for my patients it was very important to know what their day was like, what kind of work they did, what activity level they had and so on. I always asked that at the very first meeting since that became my golden ruler as to how they were doing. As I explained in Success with Heart Failure, even little things like going out to visit family or friends or attending Church can slowly go from being a regular and routine form of enjoyment to be a rare occasion when you have a little extra energy.

Here are two major ways we classify your heart failure:

- **New York Heart Association Class (I, II, III or IV)**
- **American College of Cardiology/American Heart Association Stage (A, B, C or D)**

The New York Heart Association Class, also called NYHA Functional Class or NYHA is an older classification used to rate the amount of limitation on activity a symptom caused for patients with any form of Cardiovascular disease. For heart failure patients the symptoms that limit patients are usually shortness of breath with activity/ exertion/ or even lying down to rest. Other symptoms can be fatigue or lack of energy of abdominal bloating. Once you have selected the symptom that bothers or limits you most, the next step is to decide how severe is the limitation.

For this example, let's say the symptom that limits you most is getting short of breath with activity. Starting with the worst severity, or NYHA Class IV, the shortness of breath (and, yes, we do call it SOB) is with you even at rest. And typically, not only are you aware of being out of breath at rest any minimal activity makes you even more short of breath. There is also a form of shortness of breath that develops after you lay down in bed for a few minutes forcing you to sit up or stand to get your breath. This is called paroxysmal nocturnal dyspnea, but these still are all NYHA Class IV symptoms.

NYHA Class III is slightly less severe and means you do not have shortness of breath once you are resting but small levels of activity consistently bring on the shortness. There are lots of ways to grade the amount of activity it takes to bring the symptom on such as the walking distance (feet or blocks) or the number of stairs that can be climbed or even if an incline will bring it on. I used to get a pretty good idea about what a patient's home floor plan looked like. They often could say with precision how many steps it was from the bedroom to the bathroom or the kitchen or the distance to the mailbox in the front of the house. Getting short of breath with this small amount of activity is NYHA Class III.

NYHA Class II, then is when the patient has no symptoms at rest or with mild activity but does get symptoms with "moderate" activity. Again, there are lots of ways to define moderate, and all of these assessments of activity limitation are subjective; often the patient has one perspective and their spouse or caregiver has another! However, NYHA Class II usually allow patients to get out of the house, do daily activities, and even climb a flight of stairs without a problem. In my experience NYHA Class II patients have to be watched carefully since small decreases in activity tolerance are often minimized by patients and they slowly "creep" towards NYHA Class III or IV seemingly under the radar.

NYHA Class I is obviously the best place to be and means that at the present time no symptoms are limiting them. Again, what often happens is that patients limit their activity or write any limitation off to getting older, not getting enough rest, etc. That is why real self-reflection and careful questioning is so important. As you might imagine since all of the NYHA Classes are subjective to some degree, we often assess functional capacity or the ability to do daily activities through various forms of walk or exercise tests. These really are corroborating the NYHA and also have a spot on the HF Patient Profile form.

There are two major points to make about the NYHA Classes: One is that they reflect the symptoms or symptoms a patient is experiencing at the present time. As such, a patient might be NYHA III today but with optimization of their medical therapy might be NYHA Class II or even I in a week or two. It is fluid and as I mentioned above the shifts between Classes can be very subtle. The other point however, which is why a careful assessment of NYHA Class is so important, it has been repeatedly confirmed that NYHA Class alone is related to heart function, risk of hospitalization and even survival.

The Staging System was introduced into the American College of Cardiology/ American Heart Association heart failure guidelines much more recently. I was proud to be on the committee that first introduced these 4 stages and here is what the intent was and why they are such a key component of the HF Patient Profile.

The majority of patients have a slow progression of signs and symptoms but are not initially diagnosed with heart failure until they get very symptomatic and end up hospitalized. They and their families are often shocked and terrified to hear that they have "heart failure". They truth is that they have likely been on the path to developing heart failure for years or even decades. They may have had years of high blood pressure or had a heart attack in the past or have been diabetic or had a family history of heart failure but never suspected that heart failure was in store for them.

So the Stages are a one direction progression tool that really helps you understand where you are on the heart failure path and also guides what steps you and you team should be taking to treat you and most importantly to limiting your risk of progressing to the next stage! And that is really a very important strategy, since, unlike the NYHA Classes, you do not float up and down. With the Stages, once you progress to the next level you cannot return to the lesser Stage—that door is shut.

Preparing for Your Visit

You are probably itching to get on to creating your Strategic Heart Failure care plan. That is what we will cover in the next chapter. However, like all things strategic, there needs to be an understanding of who else is on your team, how likely that are to engage with your planning, what barriers there may be, and how to win their support of your efforts.

You often need to create and activate your strategic plan in steps or bit by bit. We all have do this every day...if you ever want to convince a partner, child or associate about a plan or idea that they may not be open to, you typically find ways to build your case, make sure they see value for themselves and slowly break down opposition and often even make it seems like it was their idea! The same is true in patient and provider relationships.

I bring this up since I have encountered a few common barriers patients tell me they have encountered when trying to become engaged and empowered in helping to lead their healthcare.

And there can be a range of responses for which you have to be prepared.

For example, when you say, *"I want to review my heart failure status and see where there may be opportunities for us as a team to do ever better",* an entire range of responses, or no response at all, may result. The bottom line is to know the team members and build trust with them as they should be doing with you.

So let's walk few a few interactions you might have as you begin to be a strong partner in your Strategic Heart Failure plan. I will tell you that there is no formula to do this and success will depend upon your knowledge, your willingness to listen and learn from explanations that have never come forward before, but also use your skills of communication and emotional intelligence so that they know this is about building collaboration, trust and a win-win in every way.

Focus. Perhaps the first step is to pick the individual member of the team with whom you have the best, meaning most trusted relationship. Sometimes, when you first get referred to a heart failure team you may they may all be strangers and you have not had time enough to pick that person. That does not mean that you sit and wait, and you then, may have an opportunity to skip directly to the step, I call GOALS, below. Also, if you have been referred, you might think it best to keep your discussion with the professional who referred you since you already know them and may have a trusting relationship. Unfortunately, while this may make you, and them feel comforted it does not provide clarity to the team that will be guiding your care that you want to play an active and informed role in your care and that you are a great partner to be on the team with them. Start it off with a seat at the table if you can.

However, the most common scenario in my experience is that there is usually at least one person who is initially the face of the team for you. Often, if the team is called to provide care for you in the hospital or set up follow up in their office a nurse might be the person you meet, They might be a nurse practitioner or nurse educator or even a nurse working with the cardiac rehabilitation program. It could also be a doctor, Cardiologist or Advanced Heart Failure Cardiologist who was asked to consult on your care. Regardless of who it is the focus of the initial discussion you might want to have is on expressing the desire to work as a team, and knowing all the members of the team and their roles. (See TEAM, below).

Team. Among the things that will make you successful working with the team is know who the members of the team are, what their roles are and making sure they know your desire, actually, your expectation that they will view them as a link to the rest of the team so that you do not have to clarify to each individual member your desire to participate in your Strategic Heart Failure plan. You will also know how the team will communicate with you and who are the decision makers involved with your plan. You may be very familiar that often, and this happens commonly in a hospital setting and in teaching situations, where they may be a range of professionals from students to educators involved with your care, and they may each have an opinion about best next steps. The process hopefully allows for student learning yet allows the best knowledge to be brought to your personal situation so that you get the best care. The point is that all team members have a role but not all will play a permanent role in your care. They may be "rotating" on the heart failure service. Others may be in other forms of training where their time on the team is limited. Remember to FOCUS on one trusted team member, communicate your wishes, ask them to serve as a link to the rest of team and let them know that you are counting on them!

It is also important to provide the team members the same items you have asked of them. Make sure they know how to best communicate with you, can the call your mobile or home phone, what is the best time to reach you for non-urgent matters or even how to address you- what will build your trust and what will detract from that trust. Similarly, you make clear that you will pass along information to the family and friends you desire, or if there is a key friend or family member your like to have also receive regular updates on your care and progress.

Goals. The thing to remember about goals is that they are dynamic, they are influenced by knowledge and available options. So that if you are Stage A or B (see Heart Failure Profile) your goal might be to prevent ever progressing to having heart failure symptoms or being hospitalized. What never should change about your goals is that they are yours to share, they should be heard and not minimized. How this is best done is up to you and your team. Goal setting can occur in crisis situations such as with sudden worsening, hospitalization and goal setting around topics like device implantation, heart transplantation or hospice care. However, a major purpose, yes, a goal, of the Strategic Heart Failure plan is to allow enough insight to anticipate changes in your status and set goals aimed at stabilization and disease reversal.

Goals should be concise yet specific enough to be understood by all team members. You might think of them as a newspaper headline. The details or the nitty gritty, including what the team might tell you as to what barriers exist to make that goal less achievable are part of the CONVERSATION section below. Let me give you just one possible goal you might end of discussing with the team and then dissect it a bit in the CONVERSATION section, below.

Goal statements:

1. I read that spironolactone is can affect my survival; Is that a medication
    I should be taking?

Conversation. While this part may not take place until your actual visit, it is
good to do some preparation, or have a dry run, in order to anticipate what
might come up during the conversation. This will also put you into a better
position to prepare more questions and follow ups. Like so much in life this part
also allows you to set expectations and also be ready to manage how you feel if
those expectations are not met. I think most providers welcome questions and
participation; however, as they do not know everything going on in your mind
and life, you, too, might not feel listened to is they are distracted or rushed. The
expectation setting helps you allow for that, and in the same moment allows you
to reframe the focus, team member and goal in order to make sure you are heard.

Remember, that when you are planning to express a goal or really share anything
that is important for your team to hear and engage with you should get their
attention. I understand this is sometimes a challenge! I know that providers
stand up and begin to walk out of the room as they are still talking. There is a
Strategy for that! If you cannot get them to sit back down and listen then the
next time they come into the room begin the visit with a comment that you know
they are busy but at the end of each visit it would be helpful to you to be able to
ask any clarifying questions.

This was so important in my caring for patients that the last 3 things I said
was always "is there any other questions or anything you'd like to talk about?"
Often there would be after the first time I would ask, rarely after the second
and never after the third. When I finally felt I had listened to them, asked
about their questions and sensed that they were ready to go, then, I stood slowly
and left them room. I was also blessed enough to also have experienced nurse
practitioners in the room so that if anything else came upon the patient could get
answers and have a conversation during the same visit.

If your provider consistently does not allow your questions, quite frankly, they
are not letting you be part of the goal setting a decision making needed; you

will need to try another empowered team member...or find another practice that values the relationship with you. Trust me, you will find the right team and they will be fortunate to have you as their patient!

Using the examples above, here is how the Conversation may go, from your perspective and from the providers.

1. Spironolactone: your provider might say
    a. Yeah, you're on it...we call if Aldactone (the brand name)

(Ok, that's pretty curt but know you know)

a. You're not on it because it can raise potassium and yours has been high.

(So that should trigger a bit more conversation especially if you didn't know you had elevated potassium levels. I'd want to know how long it has been high, why is it high, what does that mean, what can be done, etc. Additionally, often patients have an elevated potassium level, but it can resolve with diet, adjusting certain supplements and so on. The point you want to get across is that is spironolactone is potentially beneficial for you that you want to take steps to see if your potassium (or kidney function) is now better so that the spironolactone could be tried). You would hope that they would also say something to make you feel included and valued, like, "I check your potassium often because it has been elevated and I will make a note to re-consider spironolactone when that level comes back. Thanks for bringing it to my attention!

In this example this goal may not resolved immediately but you can put it on your tickler or follow up list. You might want to read more about spironolactone to learn more about it before your next visit. You may want to read the product description that list the indication (reason to take it), the contraindications (reasons why NOT to take it or explore the internet for Guideline information or trials that have been done with spironolactone and patients with heart failure and a similar heart failure profile.

In other words, most steps in crafting a Strategic Plan involve a thought that gets reshaped often through a series of conversation.

What you really desire is the willingness to have the conversations, share information and be part of the process.

Despite computers and electronic records, often you and the provider working together on your Strategic Heart Failure plan offers the opportunities to have both of you supporting each other to leave no stone unturned. That is clearly one of you most important roles in your Strategic Plan.

Each of these preparatory steps are important. You may need to do them a little differently, have different timing or even different approaches. However, since the ultimate goal is your success remember this concept:

Coming together is a beginning; keeping together is progress; working together is success.

Okay team member, you are now ready to engage, participate and work with the team on your Strategic Heart Failure plan, so let's move on.

Building Your Strategic Plan (Including PRO tips)

Believe it or not you now actually have the tools to plan an informed, evidence-based plan to provide you better understanding of your heart failure and get optimal care now and as new discoveries emerge. The most important aspect has been encouraging you and training you to want to have a role in your care and in knowing how to create the Strategy to get it!

What we will now do is exactly what I did for every one of my patients, every time I saw them or spoke with them. Yes, it is repetitive, but the real fun is that it is iterative. That means that every time you review your heart failure plan it should be with what is called a beginner's mind; a fresh look at your status and well as what the options or barriers are to treatment strategies.

It is like any other planning we do. For example, with a home budget, it may look relatively dry and static from month to month, but life happens and there may be a shift upwards or downwards on the income side, there might be an incentive or bonus, or you may be laid off. On the spending side you have paid off your car so no more monthly payments, or your car has broken down and needs repair or you need to replace your car. You know how it goes...always something!

But the value of regularly reviewing your budget and thinking Strategically is to be able to plan for what might be ahead, perhaps save a little money each month and be less stressed when that unexpected expense arises. The same holds true with heart failure. For many patients their course is one full of unexpected surprises; unexpected office and hospital visits, admissions, procedures, complications, side effects, and so on. While heart failure cannot always be cured the goal is to detect it, slow down it's progression and reverse it as much as possible.

And just like a budget which may be anxiety producing to review on a regular basis, looking at YOUR Strategic Heart Failure Plan head on, which has implications about your health future, your list of medications and possibly devices and yes, even possibly your risk of hospitalization or even shortened life may not be an exciting task. In the long run, however, I believe that diving in, engaging and demanding a role in your health future will provide more satisfaction, security and sense of empowerment and much less stress.

So, let's get Strategic!

Start with the Heart Failure Patient Profile

There is a copy of this document in the Appendix of this book but is available as a free PDF download on my the book's Website (www.strategicheartfailure.com[1]) and on my Authors Page. You can also get a free PDF on this Facebook Page for Strategic Heart Failure: https://www.facebook.com/SHF2019/

The profile is really a shorthand summary of just some of the pieces of information about your that shed light on the severity of your heart failure, the symptoms you may or may not have, current damage to your heart, retention of fluid and so on. Part of your journey will be to learn this shorthand and become conversant with the terms your team already uses as a "language" to help take care of you.

When you first look at the profile you might say "I have no idea what these words or initials mean!" So let's run through them. That will allow you to begin your self-learning and exploring using the internet, medical references and even just to be able to speak the same language with you team.

Again, I am emphasizing that these are not anywhere near all the useful data points, terms, words or initials that are used in the heart failure language but these are the fundamentals, and some of the ones I think really help give a clear picture of where you are at AND what are the next steps in your plan.

If you need more detail about any of these terms, look then up or refer to Success with Heart Failure—all versions included these basic definitions.

Etiology. This means the cause of your heart failure. Sometimes we know and sometimes we have yet to find out, and we will continue to search. This is really important because know the cause often directs what is the best treatment. One example: if blocker coronary arteries is the cause then we may say "the etiology

---

1. http://www.strategicheartfailure.com

is CAD (coronary artery disease) or ischemic cardiomyopathy." One more important feature of knowing the exact cause is that it often allows being alerted to new treatments that become available for diseases like cardiac amyloid. Knowing that you had the COVID-19 virus, as another example, alerts your team to several distinct issues that may cause you to develop or worsen heart failure (see chapter 8).

Date First Known. This is the timestamp of when you first became aware of having heart failure. You may have just been hospitalized today for heart failure and had never before been told you had it. But you remember having years of high blood pressure and being told 5 years ago that your heart was a little weak. Now the dots are connecting, and you have been on this path for at least 5 years and maybe much longer.

NYHA Functional Class. This is an older classification system that has been used in all forms of heart and vascular diseases. It stands for *N*ew *Y*ork *H*eart *A*ssociation functional classification and refers to 4 levels of symptoms patients may have with 1 being no symptoms with normal activity and 4 being symptoms even while resting. It obviously is somewhat crude but over many decades has been very useful and and it evens correlates pretty well with left ventricular ejection fraction (see below, and see Success with Heart Failure for a deeper discussion). One of the downsides is that the classification does really not become applicable until someone has symptoms. (See ACC/AHA below.)

ACC/AHA Stages of Heart Failure. In 2001 I was fortunate to help write updated guidelines for heart failure. The guideline set was, and remain a standard in the US and around the world. The guidelines were the effort of the American College of Cardiology and the American Heart Association for many years and now the Heart Failure Society of America has joined in the effort. In 2001, or actually about 18 months before the 2001 date as we discussed advances we all wished for our patients with heart failure, we realized with had an enormous problem with recognizing not only early forms of heart failure but also those patients who were at a much higher risk of developing heart failure. At the time for patients who had no signs or symptoms of heart failure there no way to get a jump on the disease and try and prevent heart failure from developing or progressing. We recognized that we needed to find a way to call out that heart failure usually develops slowly, insidiously over years or decades in most cases and we needed a classification system that called this out to health professionals. This because the Stages of Heart Failure classification. (For more information see links in the appendix or Success with Heart Failure). Very briefly, it is another 4 Stage systems with A, being at risk for heart failure (family history, having diabetes or hypertension), Stage B, having some structural changes in the hearts size and function, but still no signs or symptoms, Stage C, having overt heart failure with signs and symptoms and Stage D, having advanced heart failure and having signs and symptoms despite usual treatments. At this stage there is consideration for heart transplant, left ventricular assist devices or palliative care.

MOGES. This is another classification system that is unfortunately not routinely used that looks at multiple features of an individual's heart failure and defines the shape and function of the heart (Morpho-functional), the other organs and body systems involved, the genetic linkages, the etiology and the stage. If you search MOGES you will find a very interesting page dedicated to this system. Especially as we uncover the genetic links to more and more forms of heart failure, I believe this classification system will be revitalized.

LVEF. The left ventricle is the major pumping chamber of the 4 chambered heart. And it is the pumping chamber that drives blood to the entire rest of the body. LVEF stand for left ventricular ejection fraction and ejection fraction is the percent of the blood that leaves (or is ejected) when the heart pumps compared to how much blood is in the left ventricle when it is completely filled. minus what is still in the left ventricle after it has completed its pumping. Normal is usually around 50-60%. This is often expressed as the fraction that it is: 0.50 to 0.60.

Example: LV completely filled holds 100cc of blood

LV after is ejects the blood holds 45cc of blood

Therefore it "ejected" 55cc of blood.

55/100= 0.55 So LVEF is 55%

There are so many factors that influence the LVEF moment to moment that is should never be viewed as a completely static number.

ECG. QRSd. Yes, this is a term you may be familiar with otherwise called an electrocardiogram (old term EKG). This is test that by using the hearts own electricity can provide a lot of detail about the heart size, function and its own electrical circuitry. In the past the ECG had roles in telling us about the size of the heart, whether there had been any damage as with a heart attack, what the electrical system looked like and what the heart rate was. It was useful as well to determine if a pacemaker was needed because the heart rate was too slow. We could also see if there were any irregular heart beats including atrial fibrillation. Fortunately, the ECG still does all those things and can be measured in our homes or from our wrist with "wearable" devices. However, in recent decades we learned that as the heart got damaged so did it electrical system. The purpose of the electrical system was to get the heartbeat, which start in the upper chambers of the heart to the bottom of the heart in a timely and synchronized fashion allowing the heart to beat efficiently. As we discovered more about the process of this de-synchronization we also learned more and had advances where specialized pacemakers and wires could be place into the heart and "re-synchronize" the effective coordination and pumping of the heart.

The QRSd is one of the measurements we can get from the ECG that tells us about the time delay and is called the QRS duration. QRS are standard names given to components of the electrical heartbeat. The importance is that we know that these specialized pacemakers might significantly help patients when there QRSd is above a certain number.

Now, pause here for a moment.

I know there are many more parts of the profile to learn about, but at this point, beside the etiology and date it all started you know about:

- NYHA FC
- ACC/AHA Stage
- LVEF

- ECG and QRSd

So, 4 measurements, all pretty routine. Two can be determined with a conversation.

One is from an ECG and the LVEF can be determined a variety of ways but commonly with a standard echocardiogram.

Please go to the figure 2 I have included in the appendix that is from the 2017 Guidelines.   (https://www.ahajournals.org/doi/full/10.1161/ CIR.0000000000000509) This is Table 2 in that document and describes the **Treatment of HF*r*EF Stage C and D.** I hope you will see that what the experts are recommending for patient with forms of heart failure with ejection fractions lower than normal and symptoms (about half of all patients with heart failure) is defined by measurements and terms you now know and can understand. Congratulations, you are on your way to being Strategy Masters!

Let me provide 2 other very important "PRO" tips for your Strategic Approach.

First, regarding the review of the Patient Profile data that should take place every visit or even more often as you review your personal status at home, is the need to make it deliberate. I guess its like anything else in life, we can become so familiar with the data points that it is easy to just breeze by them. I will warm you that familiarity or monotony can blunt your awareness that changes are taking place under your nose and that leads to missed early opportunities to react, reevaluate and make adjustment in your care.

Let me give you example. If you have been told about "early " heart failure or that perhaps your LVEF is 42% but you have no symptoms, you are able to work full time and so you are Stage B.

Then, on vacation that required more walking and stair climbing than you normally do and you notice getting out of breath when others in your family have not you need to pay attention to this observation. It is all too easy to write it off to eating more salt during vacation or just being out of shape. But you need to be brutally honest and ask why this happened and more importantly what does it mean and what actions do I need to take. In other words, if you don't have this crucial conversation with yourself then you will miss the opportunity to be a solid team member and bring it up at your next meeting with your team.

You make not reflect that your daily life, even on weekends is relatively sedate will rarely more than 5,000 steps taken each day. On vacation, when you were more out of breath you logged between 10,000 to 15,000 steps a day. So yes it could mean you are just not in shape or it could mean that now you ARE having symptoms with moderate activity and so you have shifed from Stage B to Stage C and your functional class is a solid II! Welcome to symptomatic heart failure.

However, your strategic goal is the understand what has happened and what can be done to limit further progression and get you back to being without symptoms at all. So you and your team may take a lot of steps but I guarantee you that your careful regular and thoughtful review of your status using the patient profile will make you aware of the changes long before your team might otherwise make those observations. YOUR OBSERVATIONS COUNT!

The last simple bit about your regular reviews of your status with the patient profile is that it should be done regularly, done deliberately and should be done in a quiet setting. I know some people function very well in noisy environments. We have all heard of surgeons who play rock music when they operate. However, in general, if you can set aside a quiet time for review and allow yourself to ask any question that comes up. Has anything changed? What would my spouse of partner say my FC is? Do I need to look up my current medications compared to the optimal doses? My grandfather always said, "it never hurts to ask questions!"

This review is so important and the need to be painfully honest with yourself reminds me to share with that even when the Patient Profile was present in the chart or electronic record I would often write out by hand the "core" elements which forced me to think about them, make sure they fit with my conversations, input from family and recent testing. I promise you that if you saw my patients charts you would find thousands of little "mini-profiles" scattered throughout. It kept me honest with myself and I believe improved the care of my patients.

Please the two mini-profiles below. Feel free to copy or print!

<u>Heart Failure Strategic Plan</u>

<u>Part 1. The Patient Profile</u>

Etiology   6 Mw

Stage VO_2

FC   ECG | QRSD

LVEF

BNP

Co – Morbids

A   A   B

Heart Failure Strategic Plan

Part II

	Short – Term	Medium Term	Long Term
Diagnostic			
Therapeutic			
Prognostic			

In the Mini-Profile, Part I, above, at the bottom, you see the letters A, A and B. This is another notation I use to make sure I do not overlook a key part of the medication strategy. There really 3 key medication groups that have been established to be lifesaving for heart failure patients, This is where our team would ask if # 1 is the patients on them, #2 are they on the target dose or as high a dose as they can tolerate, and #3 if not, why not?

The key groups are: Patients should be on 1 drug from each group

A Angiotensin converting enzyme inhibitors (ACEI)

Angiotensin receptor blockers (ARBs)

Angiotensin and Neprilysin Inhibitors (Entresto) (ARNIs)

A Aldosterone inhibitors (spironolactone)

B Beta adrenergic blockers (Beta blockers).

Finally, I'd like to provide a tip that was so important to me that I think may seem excessive but will increase your heart failure knowledge and organization remarkably. Here it is:

I not only thought of a Strategic Plan for all patients, but I envisioned the Plan in time intervals. As with any project or plan it can be broken down into a series of steps. These are usually logical but often thinking through the plan and timing of the steps is helpful. The time frames I used were "SHORT-TERM", "MEDIUM-TERM" and "LONG-TERM". The time frames could be flexible for sure. It depends on the situation. Often when patients were in the hospital the short-term covered until the time of discharge. Likewise, medium-term might be the first 3 months after the discharge which could a busy time adjusting medicines, trying new medicines or device or repeating testing to see what progress has been made.

You may already know that following as heart failure admission the risk of readmission is greatest in the first week after discharge and then within the first month and then in the first 3 months. The medium-term plan should be laser focused on understanding that the hospital admission was a marker for advancing disease and the strategic plan needs to address ALL the issues to control the disease advancement.

The long-term plan might be eventualities or future planning if the short- and medium-term plans are not successful. For example, they may include the need to evaluate the patient for a LVAD (left ventricular assist device) or for consideration for heart transplantation. Discussing the long-term plans is extremely beneficial to level setting with everyone on the team. Often, thankfully, the long-term plan does not become a reality. It is better to avoid the need for advanced heart failure care than to have it sneak up on the patient and the team.

Finally, into each period of time (short-, medium- and long-term) I would subclassify what is needed in each time frame using the headings: Diagnostic, Therapeutic and Prognostic. Basically, the diagnostic reflects pieces of information obtained from testing that may need to be ordered or repeated;

example might be a repeat potassium level, a BNP test, a blood volume assessment or updated echocardiogram.

Therapeutic refers to things used to treat a patient and might include adding spironolactone, changing to an ARNI (angiotensin receptor antagonist/ neprilysin inhibitor (Entresto, brand name), or upgrading the pacemaker to a CRT (cardiac resynchronization enabled device).

Finally, prognostics are tool that have been found useful in predicting future risk and then hopefully take actions to prevent any worsening. There are increasing numbers of powerful prognostics we use I heart failure. And often a diagnostic may double as a prognostic, such as 6 minute walk distances, or the use of a metabolic cart or cardiopulmonary exercise test (CPX) that often is used to determine need for consideration for heart transplant surgery.

Go Forward and Strategize. ACTION and TIMING

Like all things in life there are multiple phases of any project. Some excite and appeal to us more than others. Some evoke fear and worry and inhibit our actions and initial steps forward. Some involve tasks such as pulling together all of the pieces of a strategic plan. Others involve quiet thought, and other involve action. These may be actions we take or make happen, and there are actions we must rely on others to collaborate and get the actions accomplished!

And so, it is with your Strategic Heart Failure plan. Really till now you have done the heavy lifting of learning the reason and process of the plan. You have also probably put some time and effort into gathering data and organizing it into a framework that will facilitate how you come to better know your own heart failure and also have learned and organized the "heart failure vocabulary, words or phrases" into some pretty sophisticated conversations.

The next phase contains to two key words, **Actions and Timing**. Clearly the word Action indicates that now, steeped with a plan that is based on facts, supported by evidence and is truly yours, what needs to be done is to take the gaps that exist and take action to eliminate the gap, minimize the gap or at the very least understand why the particular gap cannot or should not be remedied at this time.

Notice that I said, "at this time". That gets us to the second word timing. And in fact, in the previous chapter, if you took the steps to create a plan that was broken into short, medium- and long-term timelines you have realized that, well, as they say, timing is everything. So, that aspect of your plan will guide you in figuring out, more or less, when gaps on care should be addressed. Obviously, worsening shortness of breath or more frequent episodes of low blood pressure are not gaps that go onto the long-term planning list!

What I mean is that often timing is determined by the venue or context of the situation. For example, if you have read that often heart failure patients may benefit from using CPAP breathing devices at night to sleep, you would first need to know some of the signs and symptoms of sleep apnea, which can easily be found online, or would be a question to ask at an office visit. Next, you might need to know if you have had a sleep study which can detect sleep apnea, and what your sleep score was and how your team interpreted the result and your potential need for a home CPAP unit. Or you may think that adding an aldosterone antagonist to you medications may be helpful. The steps that need to precede that is a careful review of your labs, potassium level, kidney function or even if it has ever been tried before...all really important steps to have in place before the question you have can be answered and helpful.

I realize this is all new for you—and your supporters and healthcare team. Like all transitions, slow and steady typically is better that sudden and abrupt.

As you may know from reading Success with Heart Failure, the inspiration and motivation to write the first book, and all those that followed came from just one of my patients, initially. Briefly, I met her when she was transferred to our Medical Center and told me she was there since she was told she "needed" a heart transplant. As I laid out a strategic plan for her and went through some initial steps to stabilize her heart failure, she became totally engaged and curious. She wanted to know what I was thinking, how I made decisions, what I was balancing with each decision and how I was crafting her specific plan. As she improved, she'd come to my office to read the book and articles about heart failure—the source documents. She remained my patient, friend, muse and constant challenger for the next 30 years—no transplant needed!

COVID-19 and Heart Failure

This book will be published in the shadow of one of the world major health pandemics. The amount of information that has emerged has been incredible as we study and learn about what the disease is, how to prevent spread, cure those infected and create a post-COVID reality worldwide.

Related to heart failure there are a few important statements that I can make right now. Briefly, in my opinion, they are:

- Most patients (approximately 94%) who die with COVID-19 also have 1 or more other disease and heart failure is one of the most common other chronic illnesses.
- Additionally, patients who have heart failure are a high-risk group for getting COVID-19.
- Patients who get COVID-19 often develop new heart failure.
- Patient who are found to have heart damage during a COVID-19 illness have a higher risk of dying.
- Unknown is if patients infected with COVID-19 but are asymptomatic are at risk of developing heart failure later.
- The COVID-19 virus has recently been found heart muscle cells of some patients.
- COVID-19 attacks the blood vessels throughout the body add the heart is not excluded.
- I believe we will see an increased number of heart failure patients who present with diffuse vascular disease and heart muscle disease.

Clearly, much more information will emerge. The important for those of you reading this book is to be alert...if you have been exposed, diagnosed with COVID-19 or think you many have had a "mild case" be alert for new or worsening signs or symptoms (see Success with Heart Failure). And don't forget to mention your concerns or suspicions to you team.

One last word, there has been some debate about the using of drugs that block one of the receptors in the body the control blood vessel tone and function.

These drugs (ACE inhibitors and Angiotensin Receptor blockers) have been fundamental in the treatment of heart failure patients. The concern was whether they play a facilitating role for the COVID-19 virus. As of this moment, the consensus is that patients who remain on these medications do better than those being taken off. AS ALWAYS, discuss this or any concern with your providers and teams—and ultimately this could be a very strategic decision of which you need to be engaged and weigh in upon!

What's New and Emerging

In Success with Heart Failure, at the end of each version I tried to talk a bit about all the new advances that were likely to be available to patients over the next few years. However, the advances within this field are happening in a fast and furious fashion. That is both good and bad.

Any new advance obviously is good—the bad is that often team, investigators, drug and device developers are all seeking the one single tweak that will cure heart failure. Heart failure is many things; it is insidious, serious, and for sure it is COMPLEX. We have spent the last 40 years unraveling the complex pathways ands mechanisms of heart failure. We have certainly come to the understanding that it is systemic—meaning it is not a just a heart or blood vessel disease. It affects every organ and tissue in our bodies and many of these overlapping co-morbidities serve to worsen signs and symptoms and survival for patients with heart failure. And heart failure impacts our strength, emotions and personal relationships.

So, yes, we absolutely need all the advances we can get. I just ask that these developers look towards impacting profoundly the outcomes and cost of care for the patient and society.

I also want to call out a couple of circumstances where I believe there is enormous opportunity for the patient with heart failure, well, simply gets underutilized for a variety of reasons. We often wonder why the heart failure epidemic continues to grow and many more patients will suffer with heart failure in this decade than in prior decades. I am not naïve and understand the complexities of the US Healthcare system, but I have come to believe firmly that a few items can create a positive shift in the care we deliver and the outcomes and quality of life for our patients.

Without great elaboration, here is my short list of strategies that I think should have greater penetration into heart failure care.

- Team Approach. The value of having multiple members of a care team, with different experiences and expertise all thinking with you about your care is invaluable. The requisite of course, is freedom to ask questions and speak one's voice. And once there is a plan, team must adhere to the approach until there a decision to make a change.

- Sacubitril/Valsartan (Entresto). You have likely seen magazine and TV ads about this drug for heart failure. Actually, it combines two drugs into one tablet. The evidence is strong that for most patients is offer many benefits. The barriers are several including cost. However, I believe the biggest barrier is resistance to change. Many patients may already be on one of the drugs in the combo and the switch over does not happen. The second drug in the combo is very important and the underutilization is an issue that should at least be raised. As I mentioned above most heart failure drugs are not titrated up to target doses and that too should be raised in your conversations.

- Blood Volume Analysis (BVA). Most of you have heard that heart failure causes you to retain salt and water. That is precisely true and related to the fact that any little damage to the heart is sensed by the body as not having enough blood volume to perfuse all the vital organs and tissues. This begin typically long before you ever have symptoms (Stages A and B). And this insidious retention of fluid is one of the driving forces for progression of the heart dysfunction and development of worsening heart failure. You have also heard that our bodies are composed mostly of water. That is also true—water plus proteins, like albumin create plasma. Adding in red cells (which carry oxygen) and white cells and platelets create blood. When these elements are within the circulation (heart and all the blood vessels) it is called intravascular volume. Actually, a very small proportion of all body fluid is in this intravascular space and so it is precisely controlled. If it is outside of the intravascular space it is either in the millions of cells of the body (intracellular) or if it is in between the intravascular and the intracellular spaces, it is in the interstitial space. The interstitial space is like a large reservoir to take overflow from the intravascular space. Long story short, precisely maintaining the intravascular volume is vital to healthy flow to all the organs and tissues. Doctors and nurses have worked hard to find ways to estimate this volume, but none are reliable or provide the precision needed. Since the 1970's there has been an approved test that can measure this volume along with a measurement of the red cells in your body. It is cleared by the FDA and payment for performing the test. Multiple centers in the US do the test, but many still do not. While I learned about this BVA test later in my career, I believe it can dramatically clarify the patient's status and give insights into how best to treat patients. It is being used in many other diseases including hypertension, syncope and sepsis and critical care. This is one to explore online.

I heartily suggest you attack the web and online resources with an eye towards careful, patient facing clear heart failure news reporting. I would suggest you monitor the Heart Failure Society of America's (HFSA) web site. The have a fantastic patient hub loaded with up to date resources (https://hfsa.org/patient). Also, you can join the organization as a patient or caregiver for a small annual membership fee and that way be in the know and get solid information (https://hfsa.org/membership/membership-benefits-and-categories).

Breaking News

SGLT2 Inhibitors (sodium–glucose co-transporter 2 (SGLT2) inhibitors)

I do want to say a word about this class of drugs that have been used for patients with type 2 diabetes for some time. What was noted that in patients taking certain of these drugs there was a decrease in the overall risk of developing new forms of heart disease and specifically heart failure. One of the ways these drugs work is to improve secretion of glucose by way of the kidneys. They also seem to improve getting rid of fluid in a way that is different than most commonly used diuretics. In the recent trials, we have been excited that when given to heart failure patients, with or without diabetes, they have better outcomes including reduced heart failure hospitalizations. So much needs to be worked out including whether there are patients who should not get these drugs (i.e. patients with type 1 diabetes) and will they be effective in all forms of heart failure, in other words those with preserved ejection fraction as well as those with reduced ejection fraction. You certainly will be hearing about these drugs in the days and years ahead so one more strategic decision ahead. And remember that the benefits with the SGLT2's were derived on top of all the standard heart failure medicines currently being used so the strategic approach gets more important every day!

Epilogue

In most of the editions of Strategic Heart Failure I have tried to end with some form of summation of what you have read and what work, and hopefully joys and successes lay ahead of you.

I was having a conversation with a trusted friend and I shared that I was working on this new book, Strategic Heart Failure. They were well aware of my prior books and asked me if it was an update on the prior books with some new bits and pieces. I told them how completely different this book is in approach, language and even tenor. I said, "this book is a distillation of what I have learned over a career spanning nearly 4 decades of caring and loving and learning from my patients with heart failure. But it is written as a coach, mentor and a completely "gloves off, no holds barred approach".

They paused a moment and said, "if you really want to help them, tell them what you would do if you had heart failure".

Over nearly 40 years rarely have patients asked me that, but when they do, it causes me to pause and try to consolidate my thoughts and experiences.

Unlike the strategic approach that is step by step, sequential and evolving, this question is more of a treatise or thesis that I am reluctant to propose, since it would never be totally inclusive and would end up being unfulfilling. I have said how complicated heart failure is.... the beauty of the strategic approach is that usually you only have to juggle 2 ,3 or 4 choices at a single decision point. The truth is that I would treat my friends and family exactly as I have outlined for you. In fact when people call and ask me about a themselves or a friend or neighbor, most of the time my suggestions are about going back to their team and asking the "Profile" questions. My hope is that those questions will drive the relationship into one that is based on sharing and trust and better outcomes! So, for now, let me leave you with 2 quotes, which are, in their own way, call you to action and, indeed, are strategic.

"Start where you are, use what you have, do what you can"

—Arthur Ashe

"Begin at the beginning," the King said, very gravely, "and go on till you come to the end: then stop."

— Lewis Carroll, Alice in Wonderland

Appendix

Heart Failure Patient Profile

This tool is perhaps one of the most important I have used over the years to make sure that I was not only looking and talking with the patient, but also having the hard facts right in front of me. It allowed me to perform an immediate reality check which was critical for any further decision making.

Almost all of the pieces of information that are on the profile are readily available from a conversation and a review of the medical records. However, the format itself serves as a checklist to make sure any important pieces of information that could influence a treatment decision is not missed.

And while most of the pieces are available, more often than not, they are not readily recalled, visualized, reviewed and updated at the time of care. It also is a point of discussion with patients and family members.

In short, the profile is a critical shorthand that describes an individual patients heart failure status, promotes communication and is a tool that helps make sure the patient is getting everything needed for optimal care.

It is precisely this kind of template that our teams used to summarize data quickly and share with all the team members when it came time for important discussions such as need for heart transplantation or mechanical support devices.

There is nothing absolute about what goes on the profile and it should adapt with new learning about measures that predict status, risk and outcomes. In the early days when the profile was handwritten inside the chart, I would include key information such as who was the Primary Care physician, pharmacy and even what kind of work they did as a constant reminder for me at every visit.

Explanations of each of the components of the Profile, what they mean and how to plug them in to your personal profile are found the in the Strategic Heart Failure Book and Masterclass.

(www.StrategicHeartFailure.com[1])

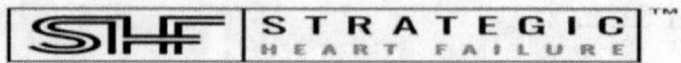

Heart Failure Patient Profile

Etiology:

Date First Known:

NYHA FC:

ACC/AHA Stage:

Heart Failure Phenotype:

MOGES:

ECG (date) Rate/ Rhythm/ QRSd:

LVEF (date):

Echo LVEDD (date):

Echo LA (date):

BNP (date):

Gal 3 (date):

ST2 (date):

CPX pVO2 (date):

CPX AT:

CPX RER:

CPX VO2/HR:

6 Min Walk (date):

4 Quadrant Position:

QOL Score/tool:

Risk Score/tool:

Key Co-Morbidity 1:

Key Co-Morbidity 2:

Key Co-Morbidity 3:

Team Members:

Occupation/Work Status:

Brief Summary:

Stages, Phenotypes and Treatment of HF

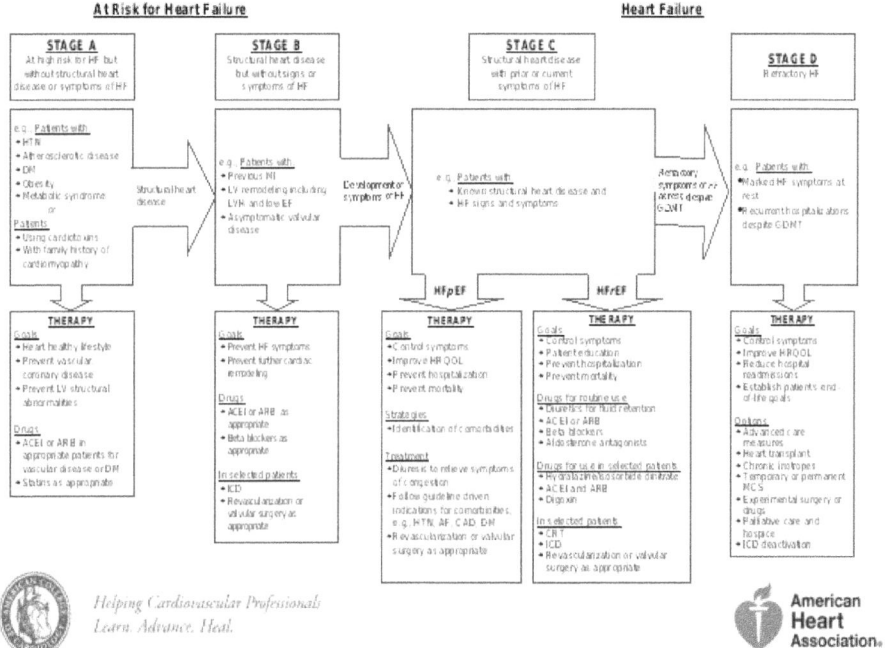

ACEI indicates angiotensin-converting enzyme inhibitor; AF, atrial fibrillation ; ARB, angiotensin-receptor blocker; CAD, coronary artery disease; CRT, cardiac resynchronization therapy; DM, diabetes mellitus; EF, ejection fraction; GDMT, guideline-directed medical therapy; HF, heart failure; HFpEF, heart failure with preserved ejection fraction; HFrEF, heart failure with reduced ejection fraction; HRQOL, health-related quality of life; HTN, hypertension; ICD, implantable cardioverter-defibrillator; LV, left ventricular; LVH, left ventricular hypertrophy; MCS, mechanical circulatory support; and MI, myocardial infarction.
Adapted from Hunt et al (38).

Recommendations for Renin-Angiotensin System Inhibition With ACE Inhibitor or ARB or ARNI

COR	LOE	Recommendations
I	ACE: A ARB: A ARNI: B-R	The clinical strategy of inhibition of the renin-angiotensin system with ACE inhibitors *(Level of Evidence: A)*,[9-14] OR ARBs *(Level of Evidence: A)*,[15-18] OR ARNI *(Level of Evidence: B-R)*[19] in conjunction with evidence-based beta blockers,[20-22] and aldosterone antagonists in selected patients,[23,24] is recommended for patients with chronic HFrEF to reduce morbidity and mortality.
		Angiotensin-converting enzyme (ACE) inhibitors reduce morbidity and mortality in heart failure with reduced ejection fraction (HFrEF). Randomized controlled trials (RCTs) clearly establish the benefits of ACE inhibition in patients with mild, moderate, or severe symptoms of HF and in patients with or without coronary artery disease.[9-14] ACE inhibitors can produce angioedema and should be given with caution to patients with low systemic blood pressures, renal insufficiency, or elevated serum potassium. ACE inhibitors also inhibit kininase and increase levels of bradykinin, which can induce cough but also may contribute to their beneficial effect through vasodilation.
See Online Data Supplements 1, 2, 18-20.		Angiotensin receptor blockers (ARBs) were developed with the rationale that angiotensin II production continues in the presence of ACE inhibition, driven through alternative enzyme pathways. ARBs do not inhibit kininase and are associated with a much lower incidence of cough and angioedema than ACE inhibitors; but like ACE inhibitors, ARBs should be given with caution to patients with low systemic blood pressure, renal insufficiency, or elevated serum potassium. Long-term therapy with ARBs produces hemodynamic, neurohormonal, and clinical effects consistent with those expected after interference with the renin-angiotensin system and have been shown in RCTs[15-18] to reduce morbidity and mortality, especially in ACE inhibitor–intolerant patients.
		In ARNI, an ARB is combined with an inhibitor of neprilysin, an enzyme that degrades natriuretic peptides, bradykinin, adrenomedullin, and other vasoactive peptides. In an RCT that compared the first approved ARNI, valsartan/sacubitril, with enalapril in symptomatic patients with HFrEF tolerating an adequate dose of either ACE inhibitor or ARB, the ARNI reduced the composite endpoint of cardiovascular death or HF hospitalization significantly, by 20%.[19] The benefit was seen to a similar extent for both death and HF hospitalization and was consistent across subgroups. The use of ARNI is associated with the risk of hypotension and renal insufficiency and may lead to angioedema, as well.
I	ACE: A	The use of ACE inhibitors is beneficial for patients with prior or current symptoms of chronic HFrEF to reduce morbidity and mortality.[9-14,25]

(Continued)

Recommendations for Renin-Angiotensin System Inhibition With ACE Inhibitor or ARB or ARNI (Continued)

COR	LOE	Recommendations
	See Online Data Supplement 18	ACE inhibitors have been shown in large RCTs to reduce morbidity and mortality in patients with HFrEF with mild, moderate, or severe symptoms of HF, with or without coronary artery disease.[8-14] Data suggest that there are no differences among available ACE inhibitors in their effects on symptoms or survival.[25] ACE inhibitors should be started at low doses and titrated upward to doses shown to reduce the risk of cardiovascular events in clinical trials. ACE inhibitors can produce angioedema and should be given with caution to patients with low systemic blood pressures, renal insufficiency, or elevated serum potassium (>5.0 mEq/L). Angioedema occurs in <1% of patients who take an ACE inhibitor, but it occurs more frequently in blacks and women.[26] Patients should not be given ACE inhibitors if they are pregnant or plan to become pregnant. ACE inhibitors also inhibit kininase and increase levels of bradykinin, which can induce cough in up to 20% of patients but also may contribute to beneficial vasodilation. If maximal doses are not tolerated, intermediate doses should be tried; abrupt withdrawal of ACE inhibition can lead to clinical deterioration and should be avoided.
		Although the use of an ARNI in lieu of an ACE inhibitor for HFrEF has been found to be superior, for those patients for whom ARNI is not appropriate, continued use of an ACE inhibitor for all classes of HFrEF remains strongly advised.
I	**ARB: A**	**The use of ARBs to reduce morbidity and mortality is recommended in patients with prior or current symptoms of chronic HFrEF who are intolerant to ACE inhibitors because of cough or angioedema.**[15-18,27,28]
	See Online Data Supplements 2 and 19	ARBs have been shown to reduce mortality and HF hospitalizations in patients with HFrEF in large RCTs.[15-18] Long-term therapy with ARBs in patients with HFrEF produces hemodynamic, neurohormonal, and clinical effects consistent with those expected after interference with the renin-angiotensin system.[27,28] Unlike ACE inhibitors, ARBs do not inhibit kininase and are associated with a much lower incidence of cough and angioedema, although kininase inhibition by ACE inhibitors may produce beneficial vasodilatory effects.
		Patients intolerant to ACE inhibitors because of cough or angioedema should be started on ARBs; patients already tolerating ARBs for other indications may be continued on ARBs if they subsequently develop HF. ARBs should be started at low doses and titrated upward, with an attempt to use doses shown to reduce the risk of cardiovascular events in clinical trials. ARBs should be given with caution to patients with low systemic blood pressure, renal insufficiency, or elevated serum potassium (>5.0 mEq/L). Although ARBs are alternatives for patients with ACE inhibitor–induced angioedema, caution is advised because some patients have also developed angioedema with ARBs.
		Head-to-head comparisons of an ARB versus ARNI for HF do not exist. For those patients for whom an ACE inhibitor or ARNI is inappropriate, use of an ARB remains advised.
I	**ARNI: B-R**	**In patients with chronic symptomatic HFrEF NYHA class II or III who tolerate an ACE inhibitor or ARB, replacement by an ARNI is recommended to further reduce morbidity and mortality.**[18]
	See Online Data Supplements 1 and 18	Benefits of ACE inhibitors with regard to decreasing HF progression, hospitalizations, and mortality rate have been shown consistently for patients across the clinical spectrum, from asymptomatic to severely symptomatic HF. Similar benefits have been shown for ARBs in populations with mild-to-moderate HF who are unable to tolerate ACE inhibitors. In patients with mild-to-moderate HF (characterized by either 1) mildly elevated natriuretic peptide levels, BNP [B-type natriuretic peptide] >150 pg/mL or NT-proBNP [N-terminal pro-B-type natriuretic peptide] ≥600 pg/mL; or 2) BNP ≥100 pg/mL or NT-proBNP ≥400 pg/mL with a prior hospitalization in the preceding 12 months) who were able to tolerate both a target dose of enalapril (10 mg twice daily) and then subsequently an ARNI (valsartan/sacubitril; 200 mg twice daily, with the ARB component equivalent to valsartan 160 mg), hospitalizations and mortality were significantly decreased with the valsartan/sacubitril compound compared with enalapril. The target dose of the ACE inhibitor was consistent with that known to improve outcomes in previous landmark clinical trials.[18] This ARNI has recently been approved for patients with symptomatic HFrEF and is intended to be substituted for ACE inhibitors or ARBs. HF effects and potential off-target effects may be complex with inhibition of the neprilysin enzyme, which has multiple biological targets. Use of an ARNI is associated with hypotension and a low-frequency incidence of angioedema. To facilitate initiation and titration, the approved ARNI is available in 3 doses that include a dose that was not tested in the HF trial; the target dose used in the trial was 97/103 mg twice daily.[29] Clinical experience will provide further information about the optimal titration and tolerability of ARNI, particularly with regard to blood pressure, adjustment of concomitant HF medications, and the rare complication of angioedema.[30]
III: Harm	**B-R**	**ARNI should not be administered concomitantly with ACE inhibitors or within 36 hours of the last dose of an ACE inhibitor.**[31,32]
	See Online Data Supplement 3	Oral neprilysin inhibitors, used in combination with ACE inhibitors, can lead to angioedema and concomitant use is contraindicated and should be avoided. A medication that represented both a neprilysin inhibitor and an ACE inhibitor, omapatrilat, was studied in both hypertension and HF, but its development was terminated because of an unacceptable incidence of angioedema[31,32] and associated significant morbidity. This adverse effect was thought to occur because both ACE and neprilysin break down bradykinin, which directly or indirectly can cause angioedema.[32,33] An ARNI should not be administered within 36 hours of switching from or to an ACE inhibitor.

(Continued)

COR	LOE	Recommendations
Recommendations for Renin-Angiotensin System Inhibition With ACE Inhibitor or ARB or ARNI (Continued)		
III: Harm	C-EO	**ARNI should not be administered to patients with a history of angioedema.**
N/A		Omapatrilat, a neprilysin inhibitor (as well as an ACE inhibitor and aminopeptidase P inhibitor), was associated with a higher frequency of angioedema than that seen with enalapril in an RCT of patients with HFrEF.[31] In a very large RCT of hypertensive patients, ompatrilat was associated with a 3-fold increased risk of angioedema as compared with enalapril.[32] Blacks and smokers were particularly at risk. The high incidence of angioedema ultimately led to cessation of the clinical development of omapatrilat.[34,35] In light of these observations, angioedema was an exclusion criterion in the first large trial assessing ARNI therapy in patients with hypertension[36] and then in the large trial that demonstrated clinical benefit of ARNI therapy in HFrEF.[19] ARNI therapy should not be administered in patients with a history of angioedema because of the concern that it will increase the risk of a recurrence of angioedema.

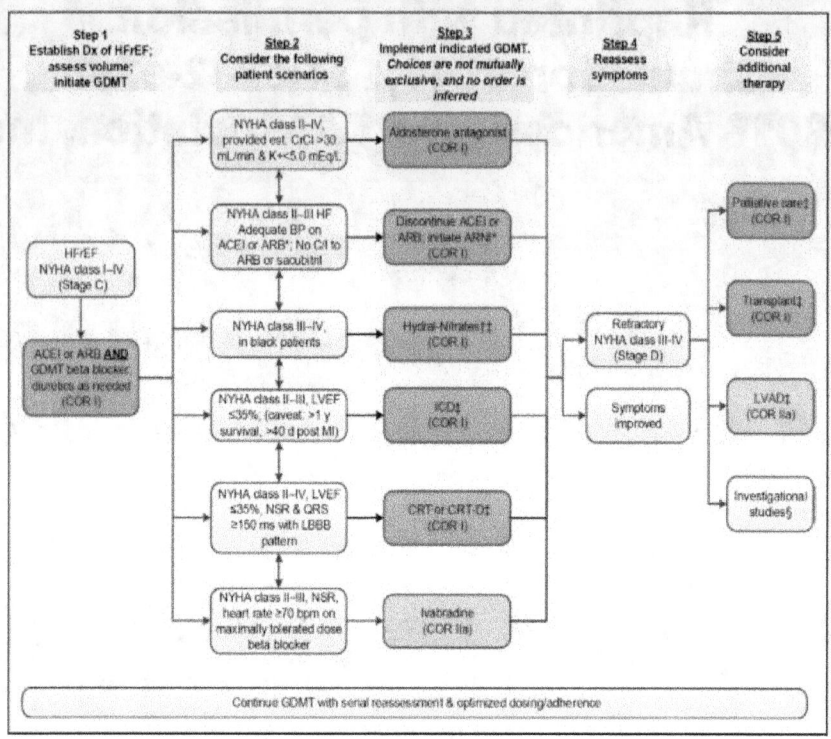

Figure 2. Treatment of HFrEF Stage C and D.
Colors correspond to COR in Table 1. For all medical therapies, dosing should be optimized and serial assessment exercised. *See text for important treatment directions. †Hydral-Nitrates green box: The combination of ISDN/HYD with ARNI has not been robustly tested. BP response should be carefully monitored. ‡See 2013 HF guideline.[9] §Participation in investigational studies is also appropriate for stage C, NYHA class II and III HF. ACEI indicates angiotensin-converting enzyme inhibitor; ARB, angiotensin receptor-blocker; ARNI, angiotensin receptor-neprilysin inhibitor; BP, blood pressure; bpm, beats per minute; C/I, contraindication; COR, Class of Recommendation; CrCl, creatinine clearance; CRT-D, cardiac resynchronization therapy–device; Dx, diagnosis; GDMT, guideline-directed management and therapy; HF, heart failure; HFrEF, heart failure with reduced ejection fraction; ICD, implantable cardioverter-defibrillator; ISDN/HYD, isosorbide dinitrate hydral-nitrates; K+, potassium; LBBB, left bundle-branch block; LVAD, left ventricular assist device; LVEF, left ventricular ejection fraction; MI, myocardial infarction; NSR, normal sinus rhythm; and NYHA, New York Heart Association.

Please follow Dr. Silver and Strategic Heart Failure at:

https://strategicheartfailure.com[2]

Also see Success for Heart Failure for more information (available on Amazon.com)

and

https://www.facebook.com/SHF2019/

For further information including Strategic Heart Failure Updates, Upcoming Masterclass Session, Live Video Sessions and Individual Mentoring Sessions.

Dr. Silver is unable to answer individual questions via email or online but does monitor the website and SHF Facebook Page.

Thank you all!

---

2. https://strategicheartfailure.com/

Don't miss out!

Visit the website below and you can sign up to receive emails whenever Marc Silver, MD publishes a new book. There's no charge and no obligation.

https://books2read.com/r/B-A-XSUK-RIOIB

BOOKS 2 READ

Connecting independent readers to independent writers.

Also by Marc Silver, MD

Strategic Heart Failure

Watch for more at StrategicHeartFailure.com.

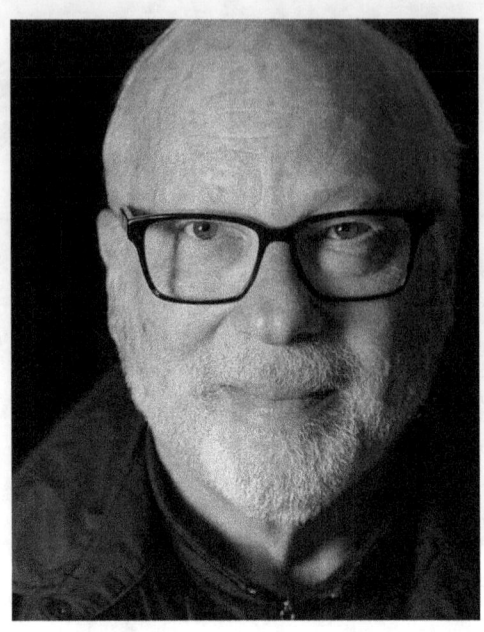

About the Author

Dr. Marc A. Silver served as the Chief, Division of Medical Services, Chairman of the Department of Medicine, and is the Founder of the Heart Failure Institute at Advocate Christ Medical Center in Oak Lawn, Illinois for 19 years, retiring in December 2017.

He is an international leader in heart failure, was a founding member of the Heart Failure Society of America, author of HFSA and ACC/AHA heart failure guidelines for over a decade, and served as Editor-in-Chief of Congestive Heart Failure for 15 years. He has authored Success with Heart Failure, now in the 4th edition.

Dr. Silver has a long-established interest in heart failure, chronic disease management and education, heart failure and multispecialty chronic disease management clinic development, biomarker evaluation and integration, integration of biometrics for early disease warning and intervention, advanced heart failure therapies including mechanical circulatory support and heart transplantation. Dr. Silver was among the first heart failure experts to receive ABIM certification in Advanced Heart Failure and Transplantation at its initial offering. In 2016 he became one of 34 Inaugural Fellows of the Heart Failure Society of America (FHFSA).He values his ability to create and grow clinical and patient care teams of excellence and meaningful, cost-conscious healthcare delivery. He has formally and informally mentored hundreds including advanced degree nursing professionals, undergraduate students seeking to explore medicine as a career path, medical students, residents, fellow and colleagues. His other passion is in linking those outside of healthcare with those inside to produce collaboration that is focused on improving healthcare safety and delivery and outcomes.

He can be reached via Twitter, Instagram and Facebook.

Read more at StrategicHeartFailure.com.

www.ingramcontent.com/pod-product-compliance
Lightning Source LLC
Chambersburg PA
CBHW071303170526
45165CB00003B/1400